MEDICAL PRACTICE MANAGEMENT

Body of Knowledge Review

VOLUME 1

Overview

Lawrence F. Wolper, MBA, FACMPE

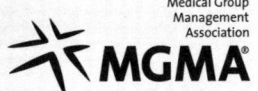

Medical Group
Management
Association

Medical Group Management Association
104 Inverness Terrace East
Englewood, CO 80112-5306
877.275.6462
Website: www.mgma.com

Medical Group Management Association (MGMA) publications are intended to provide current and accurate information and are designed to assist readers in becoming more familiar with the subject matter covered. Such publications are distributed with the understanding that MGMA does not render any legal, accounting, or other professional advice that may be construed as specifically applicable to an individual situation. No representations or warranties are made concerning the application of legal or other principles discussed by the authors to any specific factual situation, nor is any prediction made concerning how any particular judge, government official, or other person will interpret or apply such principles. Specific factual situations should be discussed with professional advisors.

Production Credits
Executive Editor: Andrea M. Rossiter, FACMPE
Managing Editor: Lawrence F. Wolper, MBA, FACMPE
Editorial Director: Marilee E. Aust
Production Editor: Marti A. Cox, MLIS
Page Design, Composition, and Production: Boulder Bookworks
Substantive and Copy Editor: Sandra Rush, Rush Services
Proofreader: Scott Vickers, InstEdit
Cover Design: Ian Serff, Serff Creative Group, Inc.

Portions of this volume were excerpted from "International Physician Practice: Historical and Cross-Cultural Perspectives on Group Practice Management" by Grant T. Savage et al., pp 12-14, and from "Physician Leadership in Medical Group Practice," by Gary S. Kaplan, MD, FACMPE, pp. 70-75 in Lawrence F. Wolper, ed., *Physician Practice Management – Essential Operational and Financial Knowledge* (Sudbury, Mass.: Jones and Bartlett Publishers, Inc., © 2005). Reprinted with permission.

PUBLISHER'S CATALOGING IN PUBLICATION DATA

Wolper, Lawrence F.
  Medical practice management body of knowledge review series : overview / by Lawrence F. Wolper ; [edited by] Lawrence F. Wolper – Englewood, CO : MGMA, 2006.
  48 p. ; cm. – (Medical Practice Management Body of Knowledge Review Series ; v. 1)
ISBN 1-56829-234-1
  1. Group practice management. 2. Practice management, Medical. [MeSH] 3. Group medical practice. [LC] 4. Medical offices – Management. [LC] I. Title: Overview. II. Medical Group Management Association. III. American College of Medical Practice Executives. IV. Series. V. Series: Body of Knowledge Review Series.

R729.5.W65 2006
658.042.W65   2005938792

Item 6465

ISBN: 1-56829-234-1   Library of Congress Control Number: 2005938792

Printed in the United States of America
10 9 8 7 6 5 4 3 2 1

Dedication

To Emily and Michael
Challenge, change, and enjoy the future.

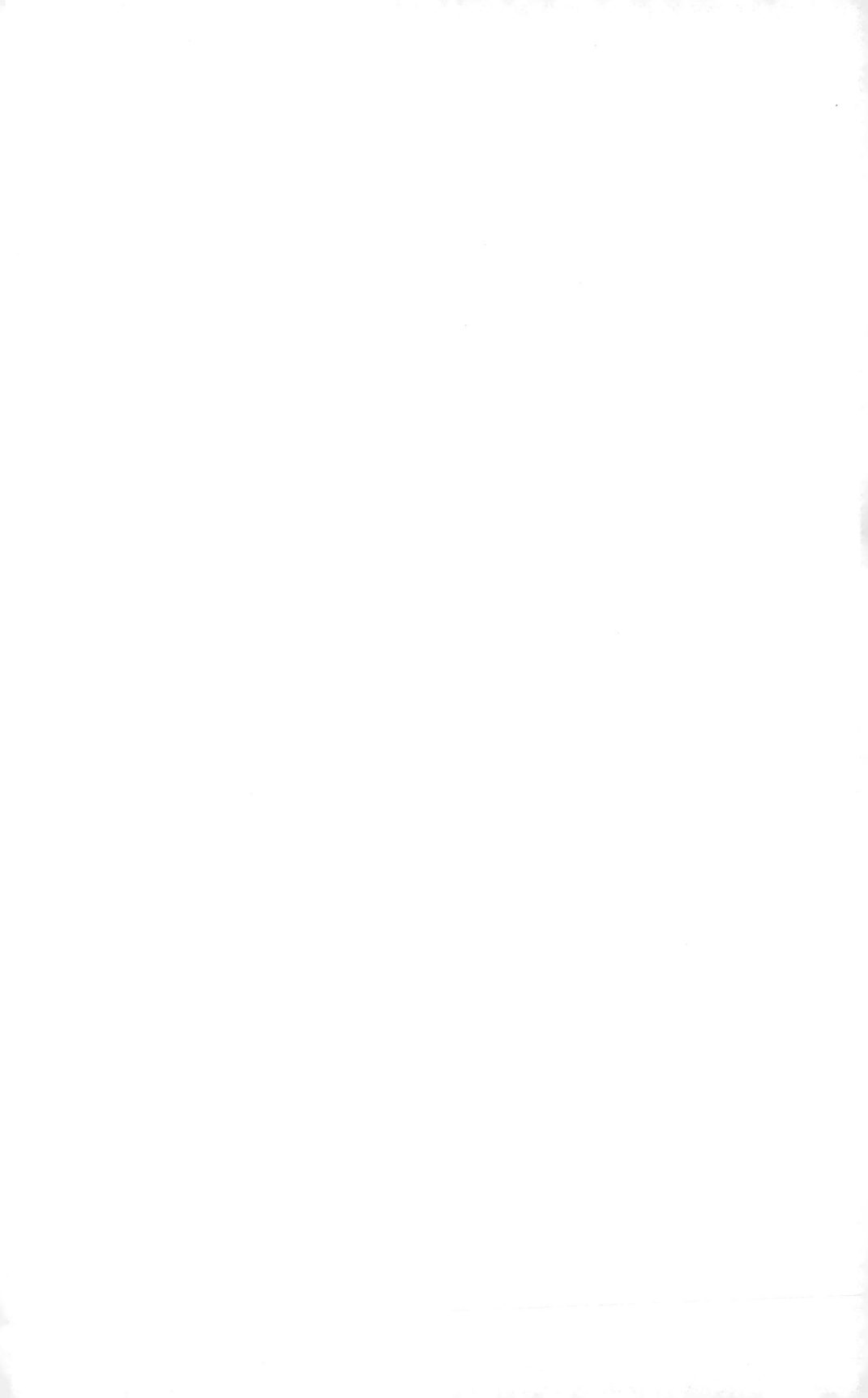

Acknowledgments

It has been a pleasure working with the principal
authors as well as the staff at the MGMA. I particularly would like to thank Marilee Aust for her
assistance, motivating ways, and the ability to
assertively push me while at the same time being
most genteel.

LAWRENCE WOLPER, MBA, FACMPE

Contents

The Development of the Medical "Group" Practice
in the United States   1

    A Brief History of U.S. Medical Practices

    Spectrum of Group Practices

Leadership in Medical Group Practices   5

    Types of Group Practices and Implications for Leadership

    Trends in Group Practice Leadership

The Medical Practice Management Profession's
Body of Knowledge   17

    How MGMA and ACMPE Use the Body of Knowledge

Overview of the ACMPE Body of Knowledge   21

    The Structure of this Body of Knowledge Series

The Body of Knowledge for Medical Practice Managers   25

An Overview of the 8 Volumes

    Business and Clinical Operations

    Financial Management

    Governance and Organizational Dynamics

    Human Resource Management

    Information Management

    Planning and Marketing

    Professional Responsibility

    Risk Management

Conclusion   39

Notes   41

About the American College of Medical Practice Executives   45

About the Author   47

The Development of the Medical "Group" Practice in the United States

THE NATIONAL LIBRARY OF MEDICINE defines medical group practice as: "Any group of three of more full-time physicians organized in a legally recognized entity for the provision of health care services, sharing space, equipment, personnel, and records for both patient care and business management, and who have a predetermined arrangement for the distribution of income." Medical group practice – which may also refer to collaborative medical work by physicians – is grounded in the social and economic, as well as the preventive and curative, practices of physicians.

Throughout most of Western history – albeit, with some notable exceptions – physicians have had solo practices. However, beginning in the 1700s and accelerating rapidly in the 1800s and 1900s, several forces radically changed not only what physicians were capable of providing, but also how and where their services could be accomplished in the United States and in Europe.

■ A Brief History of U.S. Medical Practices

Despite the growth of single- and multispecialty group practices during the 1800s, most physicians in the United

States were still engaged in competitive solo practices as generalists. Five arenas for group practices took hold in the early 1900s: dispensaries, community health centers, academic medical centers, industrial medical programs, and private medical clinics.[1] The development of each type of organization in the United States is discussed briefly here.

Dispensaries

Dispensaries are the oldest of these five practice arenas for physician groups. The first dispensary was founded in Paris in 1630 by a wealthy Protestant physician and 20 of his colleagues, all of whom agreed to provide free services for poor, sick people. As originally conceived, the dispensary was a large multispecialty group of health care practitioners that, unlike a hospital, focused on ambulatory care. In 1900 in the United States, approximately 100 dispensaries were situated in large cities. U.S. dispensaries flourished until around 1920, and their numbers then began to decline, primarily due to the establishment of short-term general hospitals, which increasingly functioned less as custodial homes and more as sites of medical treatment, and the emergence of public health clinics, which focused on personal hygiene and health education.[2]

Community Health Centers

Despite the decline in the number of dispensaries, however, the concept of the dispensary has not died in the United States. The successors to these institutions are federally qualified community health centers, which were established in the 1970s and 1980s as safety-net providers of primary care and have received renewed attention in the past few years.[3,4,5] These community health centers are typically staffed by salaried physicians, who focus on primary care (family practice, pediatrics, dentistry, and ophthalmology), supplemented by interdisciplinary teams of nurse practitioners, social workers, health educators, and others. As in the tradition of the dispensary, the focus is on high-quality care for the poor and needy.[6,7,8,9]

Academic Medical Centers

The first academic medical center in the United States was founded at Johns Hopkins University in Baltimore and spawned the establishment of similar practice groups around the country during the early 1900s.[10,11,12] The spread of the Johns Hopkins model of medical specialties, such as pediatrics and urology, solidified the notion of a multispecialty group practice.[13] Today, the 125 academic medical centers in the United States provide both medical school instruction and highly specialized care in ambulatory clinics and teaching hospitals.[14]

Industrial Medical Programs

Industrial medical programs had their roots in the industrial revolution. In the United States during the late 1800s "industry" primarily meant lumber, mining, and railroads, all of which were located in remote parts of the country. As an incentive to work for these companies as well as to ensure that employees were productive workers, company owners offered prepaid medical plans to prospective employees and hired physicians and other health care providers to deliver that care. The expansion of this type of prepaid medicine to the public, however, was opposed by many local and state medical associations.[15] Nonetheless, in 1929, Donald E. Ross, MD, and H. Clifford Loos, MD, founded the first prepaid group practice in Los Angeles. This physician group worked for about two years, serving municipal workers for a monthly price, before it was barred from the Los Angeles County Medical Society due to strong resistance to prepaid medicine.[16]

Private Medical Clinics

The first private medical clinic in the United States, established by Charles and William Mayo, had seven or eight staff members by 1900. It became a multispecialty practice early in its history with the addition of laboratory and X-ray specialists.[17,18] By 1929, the Mayo Clinic had grown to 895 staff members, 386 of whom were physicians.[19] Many of the physicians who trained at the Mayo

Clinic used the same model to establish group practices in other parts of the United States. The number of private medical groups grew rapidly in the early 1900s, especially in rural areas, where there were few hospitals.

■ Spectrum of Group Practices

Group practice has flourished in the United States under various forms for more than a century. During the early 1900s, a variety of forces influenced physicians to organize. In 1932, the American Medical Association recorded around 300 medical practice groups, averaging five to six physicians.[20] By 2003 – the most recent national survey data on group practice available – that number had grown to 19,747 medical group practices.[21]

In 1996, 70.9 percent of the medical groups in the United States were single-specialty, 22.4 percent were multispecialty, and only 6.8 percent were family or general practice groups. Specialty medical practices encompassed medical (e.g., allergy, cardiovascular diseases, dermatology, gastroenterology, internal medicine, pediatrics, and pulmonary disease); surgical (e.g., general, neurological, obstetrics/gynecology, ophthalmology, orthopedics, otolaryngology, plastic, and urology); and other specialties (e.g., anesthesiology, diagnostic radiology, emergency medicine, neurology, pathology, psychiatry, and radiology).

Depending on the type of group practice, the median size ranged from four to eight members, similar to the size of groups in the 1930s. Multispecialty groups with primary care physicians were generally the largest (mean of 27.2, median of eight physicians).[22] These trends have continued in the 2000s, with the top five specialty practices in 2003 being internal medicine, pediatrics, family practice, general surgery, and obstetrics/gynecology.[23] Moreover, between 1996 and 2003, large groups with more than 100 physicians increased their market presence, from 218 (1.1 percent of all medical groups), comprising 28.7 percent of the physicians practicing in 1996,[24] to 241 (1.2 percent of all medical groups), comprising 29.5 percent of the physicians practicing in 2003.[25]

Leadership in Medical Group Practices

ALTHOUGH MEDICAL GROUP PRACTICES have been in existence since the early 1900s, they have become much more prominent as major modes of health care delivery over the past 20 years. Physicians are increasingly choosing to practice in a group practice for many diverse reasons, and the implications of this emerging trend are significant. Physicians just graduating from training programs are increasingly choosing to practice in a group practice setting, and many established physicians are looking to become members of groups in many communities.

■ Types of Group Practices and Implications for Leadership

The spectrum of group practice types is wide, and each has unique characteristics that require varying levels and models of physician leadership. Despite different sizes and types of group practices, it is clear that effective leadership is a common and critical success factor. Therefore, ensuring that physician leadership is appropriately matched with specific group practice type and exploring optimal models of leadership for specific types of group practices are pursuits of considerable interest. Many different leadership models exist today, each with its own strengths and weaknesses. Understanding these models and the role of the physician leader, as discussed in this section, can facilitate group practice success.

Small Single-Specialty Group Practices

Smaller single-specialty groups typically have not placed a high priority on strong physician leadership. Often, a business manager or bookkeeper has assumed the oversight of billing and collections, and little attention is paid to staff development, enhancement of clinical care delivery, or teamwork. The physician leader, often the senior partner, may be called the managing partner. There is often no job description or salary designated for this role, however. These individuals may provide leadership by force of personality and seniority, and problem solving is frequently ad hoc or reactive in nature.

Maintaining the status quo and the physician income stream are felt to be key priorities for these groups, and it is only in recent years that challenges to this status quo have precipitated more formal attention to leadership roles and responsibilities. The need to become increasingly entrepreneurial has been an important factor in this recent role evolution, and many senior physician leaders in these types of groups are passing the baton to younger, more outwardly focused individuals. The leaders in these practice settings may serve in this role for only a brief period, and, in fact, leadership selection may often be on a rotational basis, leading to little continuity, a perpetual steep learning curve, and limited effectiveness.[26]

Small Multispecialty Group Practices

The small multispecialty group model presents considerable leadership challenges beyond that of the single-specialty group. Understanding the group's mix of specialties and their important roles in furthering the group's mission and strategies as well as issues of growth and resource allocation requires considerable leadership skills.

Recruitment and retention of physicians to multispecialty group practices face unique challenges as well. Some physicians are easily attracted to an environment where they work side by side with colleagues in multiple disciplines. Others feel it is critical that their primary allegiance be to their specialty; these physicians have difficulty integrating into multispecialty practices.

A major flashpoint of conflict in these settings is physician compensation, just as for the small single-specialty practice. Although the design of compensation plans in these small multi-specialty groups may fall to the manager or administrator, implementation and support for these plans are critical to their success and highly dependent on physician leadership.

Given what are likely time-limited opportunities for procedu-ralists to significantly enhance their income, the challenge to these multispecialty groups is to create and provide a value proposition that leads to recruitment and retention of highly paid specialists. Conversely, it is imperative that primary care physicians within these groups understand the significant role the proceduralists play and the need to provide market-competitive compensation. Failure to understand these important issues has led to fractionation and dissolution of many small multispecialty groups; only those groups with effective physician leadership find themselves able to survive and thrive in these turbulent times.

Large Multispecialty Group Practices

Large multispecialty group practices – those with more than 100 physicians in various specialties – are present in most urban communities across the country and in selective rural settings. They constitute many of the most prestigious group practices in the United States, and have often been led by highly visible, prominent physician leaders. Numerous historical examples show how vision-ary founders provided strong, effective leadership during the development of these group practices.

In recent years, many of the strong physician-dominated leadership structures have embraced team concepts in response to increasing complexity, economic challenge, and a realization that the model of strong physician-only leadership has many weaknesses and potential vulnerabilities. Strong physician-centric leadership models most often have a physician leader noted for his or her clinical excellence and academic credentials. Stories abound of legendary physician leaders who ruled these groups with an "iron hand." Administrators in these groups often were limited in their scope of work, with little involvement in strategy or quality improvement, instead filling the role of accountant or business manager. Critics of this model have pointed out that many physician leaders only dabble in management, are often intolerant of detail, and do not appreciate the complexities required.

Today, many of these large, multispecialty group practices have embraced a true team model of leadership, with strong physician CEOs or medical directors working closely with professional, executive-level administrators.

Issues facing these groups today have much to do with economics and capital investment. To strategically move an enterprise of significant size that is dominated by professionals requires significant investment and business discipline. Examples of challenges faced by these groups include those of information technology investment and facility expansion. Physician leadership must be engaged in this work to effectively implement the necessary change.

Consultants often serve to augment leadership in these large groups, and they can contribute to its effectiveness. These groups often, at varying times, require the full spectrum of physician leadership and management. They can either be nimble, change-oriented organizations, or group practices deeply entrenched in maintaining the status quo. The vision and performance of physician leadership often are the determining factors.[27]

Academic Faculty Practice Plans

Academic faculty practice plans present unique challenges for physician leadership, and these challenges are often functions of established structures and hierarchies. These group practices have functioned for many years as independent departments, most often led by strong department chairs who have clear control of departmental budgets and resource allocation. These structures coexist within a loosely defined medical school framework, and there often can be significant departmental rivalry. Their mission is not always clear, and tripartite objectives of patient care, research, and teaching can lead to significant conflict. The need for collaboration among departments has often not been established as a priority or critical success factor. The result is a significant lack of alignment and much variation in terms of support of mission and strategies.

Care delivery and academic endeavors are most often individual-based in these practices, and there is a mind-set of entitlement and autonomy among faculty. Leadership positions are most often attained as a result of successful academic careers, and many department chairs are those who have the longest curriculum vitae and the most publications. Many of these organizations purport to have a team leadership model; however, interviews and discussions with executives in academic settings suggest that true partnership and collaboration may actually be the exception rather than the norm. Academic prestige for physician leaders is often coupled with a clear hierarchy and what seems to be subservience on the part of administrative colleagues.

In recent years, academic medical centers have attempted to alter the dynamics of their faculty practice plans to create more responsiveness and compete with community-based practices and systems. The result has been a new awareness of the potential of strong physician leadership and willingness to tackle issues that previously were avoided. These issues are numerous and include those related to an unwieldy cost structure, a lack of horizontal collaboration between departments, and a lack of customer and marketplace orientation. The challenges are numerous, and what some have termed "academic arrogance" further promotes aversion to change. The necessity for strong leadership in the establishment of business principles and discipline is made all the more urgent by recent actions by the Health and Human Services Inspector General and other regulatory bodies and brought home dramatically by multimillion-dollar settlements following PATH (Physicians at Teaching Hospitals) audits.

Hospital-Based and Affiliated Practices

Hospital-based practices are relatively new entities that emerged as a result of the specter of health system reform in the 1990s. Many hospitals and hospital systems chose to acquire and employ physicians and physician groups. This was part of an attempt to "hardwire" market share for admissions and other hospital-based services. These initiatives seemed logical, particularly in multihospital communities where hospitals were competing for admissions from community-based physicians. Interestingly, this acquisition frenzy occurred even within communities with a single hospital and no competitors.

A major challenge to physician leaders of practices linked to hospitals is an understanding of mission, common goals, and strategies. Unlike many large multispecialty groups and integrated delivery systems, these organizations have their cultural roots and major focus within the hospital. These hospitals have functioned as workshops for physicians for many years, but have not engaged in the business and dynamics of physician group practices.

At times, it may seem like different languages are spoken by group practice leaders and hospital leaders. A lack of understanding of the differing priorities often leads to conflict. A typical challenge for hospital administrators and physician leaders is to determine the appropriate setting for specific activities, such as common procedures or imaging studies, which can be done either in the ambulatory or hospital setting. Hospital-owned physician practices attempt to avoid these conflicts, but this not always possible.[28]

Integrated Delivery Systems

Integrated delivery systems (IDSs) span the entire continuum of care; they typically have a significant presence in both the ambulatory and inpatient arenas. They are not necessarily associated with a health plan or financing vehicle. Physician leadership of these entities requires sophisticated levels of expertise in a wide range of disciplines. By focusing on the entire continuum of care, these systems believe they are able to offer patients optimally coordinated care for both routine primary care as well as the full spectrum of complex specialty and critical care services.

The synergies created by this model are numerous, and many of the traditional conflicts that occur between hospitals and physicians are avoided. Many of these delivery systems serve as so-called "academic halfway houses," providing academic opportunities not found in most group practices, and they do so without the structural encumbrances often present in academic settings. These practices face significant capital challenges in order to fully capture the opportunities inherent in their model. Physician and nonphysician leadership is crucial to the success of these organizations, and many have a long tradition and history of strong physician leaders. Some of the most evolved team leadership models exist in these organizations because of their complexity and the vast array of skills required when providing effective leadership and management.[29]

■ Trends in Group Practice Leadership

Group practices are increasingly recognizing the value of effective leadership. The case for strong leaders is becoming compelling, and formalizing the role of physician leader in groups of all sizes and types is becoming the norm. Resources are more readily being allocated to leadership training, development, and forming the role of leader in a way that allows significant progress to be made within individual practices. Formalization of teams and a team leadership structure characterizes some of the most forward-thinking group practices across the country. Recognition that leaders bring much to the table but cannot accomplish group practice objectives alone has led to a willingness to embrace administrative support and partnership. Strong administrative executives have chosen to work collaboratively with physicians in the group practice setting. These partnerships between physicians and administrators become even more compelling given the complexity of today's business and clinical environment. It is often difficult to separate the clinical area, with its emphasis on quality and safety, from the business and efficiency components of the group practice. Recognition that a clear understanding of both domains is important, coupled with the realization that this can best be accomplished with high-performing teams, suggests a preferred group practice leadership model for the future.

Physician Leader as Change Agent

An increasingly important role for the physician leader is as the sponsor of major change efforts. It is no surprise that in an increasingly turbulent environment, significant change is required. This is challenging even in stable environments, and during times of instability and environmental change, there is clearly a tendency on the part of physicians and other professionals to work hard to find ways to maintain the status quo. There are many compelling reasons for necessary rapid change, including quality and safety imperatives. In addition, the economic adversity faced by most group practices necessitates significant changes in the way practices do their work and the processes involved in patient care delivery. Leading these change initiatives is perhaps one of the most challenging and uncomfortable roles for the physician leader.

Numerous examples of successful change leadership exist in many industries, including health care and the group practice setting. Likewise, numerous stories and vignettes point out large-scale change that has not been successful, often due to failures of leadership. Physician leaders today must be students of change management and understand the complex organizational and individual issues that inherently promote resistance to change. Many of these issues are emotional in nature, and yet emotionally driven resistance to change can derail the most logical and fundamental change efforts.

John Kotter's books *Leading Change* and *The Heart of Change* have become increasingly popular. The constructs he describes can be utilized in many industries, including health care.[30,31] The applicability and relevance of his eight stages of successful change are readily apparent:

1. Establishing a sense of urgency;

2. Creating the guiding coalition;

3. Developing a vision and strategy;

4. Communicating the change vision;

5. Empowering broad-based action;

6. Generating short-term wins;

7. Consolidating gains and producing more change; and

8. Anchoring new approaches in the culture.

The eight-stage process of facilitating successful major change appears to be in many ways designed for the ongoing and required changes in health care.[32] Many group practices do indeed face a time of significant urgency. Marketplace realities, the regulatory environment, and concerns regarding safety and quality contribute to a sense of crisis. Guiding coalitions take many forms within medical groups, and the challenge to leadership is to create a guiding coalition for positive change. Unfortunately, guiding coalitions to resist change can be prominent and all too often assume disproportionate power.

The importance of a coherent vision and strategy cannot be overemphasized. Physicians, like all staff, need to understand the strategic direction and their role in furthering strategic objectives. This is critical for physician leaders. Once that vision is understood, they need to articulate that vision repeatedly, using all possible means. This requires a strong leadership team and often a network to "spread the word." Implementing change requires broad-based action, and physician leaders rarely, if ever, can accomplish this alone. Building broad-based support and then empowering others is critical. Piloting change initiatives in distinct areas of the group practice can generate short-term wins, which provide a foundation for further change and build momentum.

Finally, as Kotter points out, changes must be anchored within an organizational or group practice culture. This is often more difficult than it seems; the adage that "leadership culture" becomes the organizational culture is true in physician organizations as well. Clearly, the role of the physician leader in designing, managing, and implementing change is crucial to organizational success.[33]

Skills, Knowledge, and Competencies – The ACMPE Body of Knowledge

Formalization of the physician leadership and management role in group practices is a relatively recent occurrence and has not been fertile ground for research or analysis. Therefore, research leading to delineation of the leadership and management skills that are critical to success as a physician leader is relatively new. Much of what has been described is based on various authors' personal experiences, as well as anecdotal observations. This field is rich for potential research and subsequent curriculum design based on research findings. This section explores some of the available data, and addresses leadership and management competencies, styles, and implications for developing future leaders.

In 1996 and 1997, the American College of Medical Practice Executives (ACMPE), the professional development and credentialing organization affiliated with the Medical Group Management Association (MGMA), conducted a study designed to identify the roles and knowledge requirements critical to competent job performance for physician leaders and professional administrators. ACMPE also examined the relationships between these professionals and the implications for organizational change.

This study was commissioned, in part, due to the perception by ACMPE that physicians were taking on new and increased leadership roles in group practices. The research inquiry was generated by the increased complexity of the health care delivery system and a need to better understand the required competencies to ensure that necessary leadership was in place.[34]

The initial study brought together a panel of experts in medical practice administration. These were predominantly administrators who came from a variety of practice settings and had differing educational levels and years of experience. This panel examined specific performance domains, as well as the specific tasks involved in each area and the knowledge, skills, and abilities required to accomplish them. The second phase of the study involved questionnaires based on the identified domains and tasks. Analysis of the questionnaire results included a comparison of the responses of varying subgroups, including physicians and nonphysician respondents.

The study identified eight overall domains or areas of responsibility for group practice administrators:

1. Financial management;

2. Human resource management;

3. Planning and marketing;

4. Information management;

5. Risk management;

6. Governance and organizational dynamics;

7. Business and clinical operations; and

8. Professional responsibilities.

Specific skills or abilities making up each domain were then identified, and the resultant study provided a helpful framework for examining roles and performance requirements of medical practice leaders.

Among the several key findings was a general agreement on the competencies required of medical practice administrators and physician leaders. Study participants agreed that their roles as physician and nonphysician leaders were very broad, but recognized the requirement for very specific skills and abilities in a number of key areas. Although each domain received high rankings in terms of importance from both administrators and physician leaders, specific activities within the domains and the proportion of time allocated to these activities were not uniform, reflecting different prioritization. Subsequent focus groups were quite helpful in this regard.

Domains that both physician and nonphysician leaders believed to be the most critical were:

1. *Financial management*, including budgeting, accounting systems, financial analysis, control systems, financial systems, cost statements, costs of operations, third-party contracts, and retirement planning and investments.

2. *Business operations*, including operational planning, staffing schedules, ancillary support, facilities planning and maintenance, patient flow processes, accreditation, and process improvement.

3. *Human resources*, including compliance with federal and state regulations, formulation of compensation and benefits programs, the creation and maintenance of job descriptions, and employee appraisal systems.

Survey respondents also noted that governance and organizational dynamics, including change management, oversight of quality improvement efforts, governance systems, stakeholder relationships, and physician and staff teamwork, required disproportionate time and energy. One would suspect that if the survey were redone, in the current time frame, these areas might take on even more criticality.

Subsequently, four focus groups of physician and nonphysician administrators convened to review this and other studies related to competencies. Interesting findings included the higher ranking by physician leaders on the tasks within the Governance and Organizational Dynamics domain related to "ethical decision making and social responsibility." Similarly, administrators ranked "facilitating and managing change" within the Governance domain much higher than did physicians. This higher ranking on change management by nonphysician administrators was not surprising to the focus group participants. They saw leading change as a particularly difficult role for physicians; physician leaders often fear being labeled as "one of those administrators."

It was also noted that "nothing can change without physician support." Other focus group participants stated that ethical and quality issues are often used by physicians as very powerful excuses for halting change efforts. Change management is an area in which administrators can significantly help physician leaders to gain necessary skills and confidence. This has significant implications for physician–administrator team models of leadership.[35,36]

The Medical Practice Management Profession's Body of Knowledge

THE IDENTIFICATION AND ARTICULATION of a relevant body of knowledge are essential steps in any profession's development. Possession of a body of knowledge is one way that professionals establish their claim to expertise that deserves recognition. The validation of a body of knowledge by a community of peers is the prerequisite for the presentation of a profession's requirements for knowledge and skills. Changes in a profession's body of knowledge are not only expected but indicate its vibrancy.

For medical practice professionals, the ACMPE Body of Knowledge for Medical Practice Management represents just such a milestone. The validation process has provided an accurate and detailed description of the role and responsibilities of medical practice managers, the general competencies of the profession, and specific knowledge and skills for carrying out these competencies. This Body of Knowledge is a current but evolving resource that practitioners can visit and revisit for the perspectives they need to understand the foundations of their current work as well as the future challenges.

The presumption that there is a body of knowledge that practicing medical executives must master has been evident in the literature of the profession for many years.

However, the profession had lacked a clearly identified inventory of current competencies scientifically validated by the broad community of medical practice executives. To this end, as stated in the previous chapter, the ACMPE began a study in the late 1990s to identify and validate the roles and knowledge requirements for medical practice management professionals.

As part of this process, ACMPE convened a role delineation panel of experts in medical practice management drawn largely from the ACMPE membership. The 12-member panel represented a variety of practice settings, geographical regions, educational levels, and years of experience. The panel identified eight major performance domains (i.e., areas of responsibility), a variety of key tasks associated with successful performance in these domains, and the knowledge, skills, and abilities required for completing each task.

The identification of these domains and tasks was validated by a psychometric and quantitative review of the survey responses of a statistically valid sample of ACMPE and MGMA members, including physicians. Subsequent to this survey, ACMPE convened panels of subject matter experts drawn from the MGMA assemblies and societies and the Education/Information Center committees to further develop knowledge and skill statements within each performance domain.

The focus is on two main questions: What does it take to be an effective medical practice executive? What is the core body of knowledge required for proficiency in medical practice management in today's health care environment? The eight-volume *Medical Practice Management Body of Knowledge Review Series* answers these questions and more.

■ How MGMA and ACMPE Use the Body of Knowledge

MGMA, as a professional membership association, has adopted the ACMPE Body of Knowledge for Medical Practice Management as its primary source for *identifying the professional development needs of medical practice executives*. It uses the Body of Knowledge as a basis for developing and classifying a variety of education, information, and networking resources uniquely relevant to the needs and specific job duties of the medical management professional.

ACMPE uses the Body of Knowledge to develop assessments, examinations, and other resources for the professional certification process. Just as a blueprint guides the construction of a building, so a clear statement of the knowledge, skills, and abilities required for professional competence determines the content and form of an examination.

This reliance on the Body of Knowledge ensures a demonstrable link between the profession and the education, information, and certification testing that these associations provide to the practicing professional.

Medical practice management professionals at all career stages can use the information in this series to help guide their personal growth and development, as well as to advance their organizations.

In addition, physicians, planners, human resource managers, educators, and others with responsibilities for supporting the effective management of medical practices will also find this information useful for developing staffing models and management structures, creating relevant educational offerings, and establishing medical practice business goals.

To download a free copy of the *ACMPE Guide to the Body of Knowledge for Medical Practice Executives*, visit the ACMPE section on the MGMA Website at www.mgma.com/acmpe/bokguide.cfm.

Overview of the ACMPE Body of Knowledge

THE FIVE GENERAL COMPETENCY AREAS in the Medical Practice Management Body of Knowledge include:

1. Professionalism;

2. Leadership;

3. Communication skills;

4. Organizational and analytical skills; and

5. Technical and professional knowledge and skills.

Professionalism – Professionalism has been at the center of the development of medical practice management over the years. To keep pace with the emergence of ambulatory care and physician practice as the major loci of caregiving in the nation, practice managers must learn and execute management techniques in a variety of business areas, at the same time recognizing that the primary role of a physician practice is to provide accessible and high-quality care. Demands for ethical decision making, a broad and deep knowledge and skill base, and lifelong learning to function competently as a practice executive certainly place this role at a professional level.

Leadership – The emergence of the role of professional practice executive creates a corresponding requirement to lead. Leadership takes many forms. Internal leadership is the ability to distill complex management problems and solutions into readily understandable management initiatives that are designed to create change. It also requires the ability to set the tone that enables supervisory staff and physicians to assist in changing the organizational setting so that the practice operates efficiently and profitably. Leadership is also an external function. By participating in local, state, and national politics that influence regulatory change, exchanging professional knowledge among one's peers, and conveying new knowledge back to one's practice cohorts, the practice executive displays leadership that benefits the individual practice, as well as potentially changes the regulatory landscape within which all practice executives must work.

Communication Skills – The ability to absorb information and to present it clearly and concisely, in both written and oral forms, is a skill of great importance to executives in any industry. The health care industry has become, and will continue to become, more complex, and practice executives will be called upon to communicate information from a variety of specialty areas such as information systems, finance, accounting, pension and benefits, and human resource management, among many others. This broad palette of regulation and complexity may be unique to the health care industry, specifically the management of physician practices, in which individuals are required to have a particularly broad range of knowledge. Dealing with the complexities of an industry and communicating them effectively is much easier for a multimillion-dollar corporation than even a large physician practice. In many respects, therefore, more responsibility falls on the shoulders of practice executives to stay abreast of information, be agents of change, and effectively communicate these changes to physicians and others.

Organizational and Analytical Skills – In addition to the requirement to stay abreast of a range of specialty skill areas, the practice manager is required to have a sound understanding of organizational theory and practice. Decisions in medical practices do not always conform to the manner in which they occur in large organizations and corporate America. Physicians are not only owners in the practice, but they also are the caregivers as well as stakeholders in the manner in which the practice is managed. Therefore, they typically are involved in practice management and the establishment of policies and procedures. Understanding the organization and decision-making structure of a practice is instrumental to success.

Analytical skills in any practice are critical to monitoring change, assessing the financial status of the practice, monitoring billing and collections, and making decisions of magnitude. Without these skills, the effectiveness and professional growth potential of the practice executive are limited.

Technical and Professional Knowledge and Skills – A wide range of skills and professional knowledge is required of the practice manager. The eight performance domains defined by the ACMPE Body of Knowledge define areas of technical and professional knowledge and skills that the practice manager should acquire.

- Financial Management
- Human Resource Management
- Planning and Marketing
- Information Management
- Risk Management
- Governance and Organizational Dynamics
- Business and Clinical Operations
- Professional Responsibility

These eight areas of technical and professional knowledge and skills have long formed the basis for Certification and Fellowship in the American College of Medical Practice Executives, and also are the basis for most publications, seminars, and assessments developed by MGMA and ACMPE.

■ The Structure of This Body of Knowledge Series

Each of the volumes in this series expands upon the eight domains listed above. The *ACMPE Guide to the Body of Knowledge for Medical*

Practice Management serves as a detailed outline of the required competencies, and this series presents greater explanatory information to help readers master key tasks within each of the domains. Within the volumes, case studies or vignettes demonstrate the practical application of the tasks being discussed. In addition, the volumes offer sample questions derived from the subject matter that are representative of questions posed in the written portion of the ACMPE Board Certification examinations.

Readers wishing to pursue greater levels of substance and detail are encouraged to read *Physician Practice Management – Essential Operational and Financial Knowledge*, Lawrence F. Wolper, ed., (Sudbury, Mass.: Jones and Bartlett Publishers, 2005).

The authors for the *Body of Knowledge Review Series* were chosen because of their demonstrated knowledge of the subject and its specific applications to the management of medical practices. Many are Fellows or have obtained Board Certification in ACMPE. Others are leaders in the industry and noted professors.

The Body of Knowledge for Medical Practice Managers

AN OVERVIEW OF THE EIGHT VOLUMES

■ *Business and Clinical Operations –*
Edward Gulko, MBA, FACMPE, CHE

Some of the 10 key tasks that comprise this Body of Knowledge performance domain are business functions only, others are principally clinical functions, and some represent an overlap between the two. The medical practice executive's responsibilities likewise sometimes involve business plans, sometimes clinical matters, and often a combination of the two.

Task 1, facilitating business operations planning, is an outgrowth of strategic planning because the executive's stewardship of operations, structure, and staffing must be consistent with the practice's vision, mission, values, and long-term goals. The administrator is expected to develop an understanding of staffing analysis and scheduling and the underlying issues such as the proper number of staff and physicians, the applicable skill mix, and the standardization of human resource policies that address employee concerns, all encompassed in Task 2. Task 3 addresses the analysis required for the executive to identify opportunities to add ancillary services such as X-ray, pharmacy, rehabilitation, and laboratory, among others.

These services not only represent potential sources of revenue, they also are designed to provide comprehensive services to patients, and to do so in a patient-friendly manner. Supplies and equipment are the tools that physicians and staff need to function efficiently from day to day. When equipment breaks down, or supplies are unexpectedly expended, the patient care process breaks down.

Task 4 requires the administrator to develop procurement and inventory control systems that are designed to minimize the adverse impact of equipment failure and out-of-stock supplies. In fulfilling Task 5, facilities planning and maintenance programs, the administrator must address facility design as it relates to physician/staff workflow, patient safety, and federal and state compliance. In addition, this task touches on the many facets of facility management including fire drills and evacuation, housekeeping standards, utility requirements (heating, ventilation, and air conditioning, or HVAC), and the policies and procedures of the Occupational Safety and Health Administration (OSHA) and the Americans with Disabilities Act of 1990 (ADA).

Task 6, establishing patient flow processes, addresses one of the most important success predictors in a medical practice. In performing this task, the medical practice executive evaluates and manages the practice's daily flow, including emergencies, queuing, cancellations, no-shows, and barriers to process. The key patient flow issues regarding business requirements, such as patient encounter management, physician time maximization, treatment plans, informed consent, referral processes, patient access, and confidentiality, are all part of the purview of this task for the medical administrator. Task 7 focuses on the medical practice executive's role in developing and implementing patient communications systems. Centralized call centers and telecommunications software and hardware have made it much easier for staff to manage patient appointments, oversee the efficiency of operators, decrease patient no-shows with automated appointment reminders, and so forth. Better handheld devices enable physicians to communicate more efficiently with their offices as well as with colleagues with regard to patient care matters. Quality lies at the heart of the contemporary practice.

Task 8 covers the development of data models for clinical pathways and clinical outcomes. More specifically, the practice administrator must be familiar with the use of multidisciplinary teams; the impact of redundancy; external agencies and payers; quality assurance programs; chart review; and evaluating physician, payer, and patient satisfaction data. Closely related to the prior task is Task 9, relating to the administrator's ability to monitor systems for licensure, credentialing, and recertification. This task addresses the issues that are related to safety and health procedures, facility design and safety, quality assurance reviews, and physician and staff credentialing. Lastly, the administrator should develop ongoing processes for continuous monitoring and improvement of clinical operations, the focus of Task 10.

■ Financial Management –
David N. Gans, MHA, FACMPE, and
Lee Ann H. Webster, MA, CPA, FACMPE, et al.

Within Financial Management, the largest domain in the ACMPE Body of Knowledge, are 12 tasks that the practice manager must carry out. Task 1, the preparation and management of budgets to achieve organizational objectives, is the underlying mechanism used by the administrator to measure the operating performance of a practice. By using assumptions based on the strategic plan, the practice executive should prepare both revenue and expense budgets for the coming year and evaluate whether the practice is achieving its plans on a monthly basis. The annual operating budget also is utilized to prioritize projects to be consistent with the financial goals of the practice and to allocate capital and human resources in such a manner as to best achieve the goals of the practice.

All revenue/cash transactions must be handled properly to avoid misallocation and occasional theft. Even in the smallest practices, developing internal accounting and financial management controls (Task 2) is crucially important. Internal control manifests in many ways, but the most frequent application of internal control has to do with the integrity of data and control over payment and expense transactions.

By performing Task 3, preparing financial statements and conducting financial analysis, the administrator assures that accounting for revenue, expense, liability, and assets in a practice is performed and reported in a consistent and accurate manner. One of the most important uses of the operating budget, as expressed in income statements, balance sheets, and cash flow statements, is to communicate complex financial information to key stakeholders such as the board of directors, shareholders, and to key managers in the practice. The communication of this information is also done through the use of benchmarking and ratio analysis. These tools distill complex information to easily understood benchmarks, many of which can be compared to regional or national operating data.

Through Task 4, developing and managing material procurement and payment systems, the practice executive has the ability to control inventories, and to identify when materials should be purchased by the practice.

Task 5 – developing coding and reimbursement policies and procedures to maximize cash flow – addresses the administrator's responsibility to manage the practice's revenue stream. The administrator must be intimately familiar with the many reimbursement methodologies and systems available to the practice, such as coding systems, guidelines, and resources (resource-based relative value scales, or RBRVS; current procedural terminology, or CPT; and the International Classification of Diseases, or ICD-9), as well as accounts receivable systems, regulatory agency guidelines, and mandates.

Every practice plans for the future; to help with that mandate, the administrator is often responsible for facilitating investment planning, management, and compliance (Task 6). From financial markets and investment alternatives, the administrator can steer the practice toward or away from investment options and cash tools, and help establish the practice's investment philosophies and goals – all the while considering liquidity, risk, and return. Feeding directly into the philosophy and management of the practice's investments is Task 7, establishing business relationships with financial advisors. The practice executive must know the basics of banking, finance, accounting, auditing, and investing. In addition, the advisor relationships established within and for the practice are often handled directly through administration, and the methods for choosing a banker or investment broker should be clear.

Task 8, establishing fee schedules for physician services, is most likely the most important part of an administrator's duties. The administrator helps to establish which fee schedule methodologies the practice will follow, set charges, establish risk agreements, and use operational data sources to weight averages and count frequency. In addition, this task is performed while keeping in mind antitrust, fraud and abuse, payer and patient mix, and noncovered services.

Much has been written in the popular press about Task 9, the negotiation of third-party contracts. The ability to engage in these types of transactions is important to the success of a practice. Certain areas of the country, in which large multispecialty or single-specialty practices dominate or that are the highest in clinical performance represent a greater opportunity for the administrator to negotiate favorable rates. Relating directly to this is Task 10, developing reconciliation systems for third-party payer reimbursement. The ability to establish, manage, review, and amend accounts receivable is no small task. The administrator must identify reasons for nonpayment; develop rejection codes; track and collect withholds; appeal denials and track their rates; and collect late payments, penalties, and interest from nonpaying accounts.

In many organizations, the practice executive plays a major role in Task 11, the facilitation of retirement planning for the physicians in the practice. Outside assistance generally is necessary due to the complexity of plans and many regulations regarding retirement planning. The practice manager must have an understanding of this technical area to effectively communicate this information and make decisions regarding the most effective pension vehicle(s) for the physicians and nonphysicians in the practice.

The last task in the Financial Management domain, Task 12, maintaining compliance with tax laws and filing procedures, is one that the administrator must have under control. The responsibility of keeping the practice current on all federal and state tax payments is immense and is a key component in staying compliant and above reproach.

■ *Governance and Organizational Dynamics –*
Stephen L. Wagner, PhD, FACMPE

Notwithstanding the importance of all of the domains in the Body of Knowledge, at the core of every medical practice is its organizational governance coupled with business and clinical operations. Administrators must carry out effectively the seven tasks within the Governance and Organizational Dynamics domain.

Task 1 addresses the responsibilities and requirements of the administrator as change agent to lead and manage the organizational change process. The use of problem-solving and conflict-resolution techniques to create energy and motivation for change are presented as critical skills in this process. This task also requires the ability to guide the practice's physicians and staff through negotiation and decision making to reach consensus on important issues while maintaining trust and relationships with key stakeholders.

As the introduction to Task 2 states, constructing and maintaining the organization's governance system should begin with a clear understanding of what the process of governance entails and what the role of governance is or should be. Guided by the practice's mission and values statement, the administrator leads the organization through analytical processes to determine the most appropriate governance structure for the size and culture of the practice. Through Task 3, evaluating and improving governing bylaws, policies, and processes, the administrator strengthens that structure for the proper operation of the group and prevention of legal jeopardy. The role of the board of directors and the manner in which board decisions should be made are key components in this task.

Once the structure is in place, keeping a finger on the pulse of key stakeholders is an important element in making management decisions and adjustments. By using assessment and survey tools to obtain important data on stakeholders, situations, and personalities, the administrator addresses Task 4, conducting stakeholder needs analysis and facilitating relationship development. This understanding and analysis becomes an important basis for the remaining Governance and Organizational Dynamics tasks.

Through Task 5, the focus is on the administrator's ability to facilitate staff development and teaming by sustaining trust and constructive relationships so that staff will be motivated to work together to accomplish the long-term goals of the practice. By carrying out Task 6, facilitating physician understanding of good business practices, the administrator becomes the teacher and provides continuous opportunities for physicians to learn how good businesses operate through structured learning sessions and best practices education. With the right governance structure and constructive working relationships and dynamics in place, the organization is positioned to realize its purpose for existence – the provision of quality patient care. Through Task 7, developing and implementing quality assurance programs, the administrator focuses the attention of governance to invest in quality improvement through such monitoring activities as satisfaction surveys, benchmarking, and accreditation.

■ *Human Resource Management* –
Michael A. O'Connell, MHA, FACMPE, CHE

The Human Resource Management domain deals with the vast array of employment issues and laws as well as various management techniques such as employee handbooks and supervisory training to assure compliance. Task 1 addresses the comprehensive treatment of compensation design and benefits programs. As physician practices get larger through internal growth or mergers and acquisitions, the comparability of compensation and benefits becomes more important to attracting talented staff.

At the core of the human resources function of every organization is Task 2, establishing job classification systems and crafting detailed position descriptions. Arising from the position description is the administrator's ability to compare job functions, as well as the ability to conduct regular operational audits to assess whether employees are performing at a level that is consistent with that identified in the position description.

Through Task 3, developing employee placement programs and facilitating workforce planning, the administrator addresses the evolving human resource needs of the practice to fulfill its strategic plan and assure that the practice attracts and retains the most qualified candidates for new and vacant positions. This system allows a better understanding of the dynamics necessary to have a workforce that meets the demands of the marketplace.

Also stemming from the position description is Task 4, developing employee appraisal and evaluation systems. In addition to crafting unbiased evaluation forms, the practice also needs to assess whether employees are performing the tasks in the position description and accomplishing the goals set forth in their annual performance plans. In addition to hiring the right staff, administrators are responsible for developing and implementing employee training programs (Task 5) to keep existing skills current and to teach new skills. Training can be accomplished by sending employees to seminars given by outside organizations, by collaborating with other practices and conducting internal training, and, if the practice is large enough, by sponsoring one's own training programs.

Through Task 6, establishing employee relations and conflict resolution programs, the administrator puts into place the necessary programs and resources to help employees and management resolve issues that prevent successful accomplishment of the organization's goals and objectives. To assure that employees are treated fairly and to mitigate legal risk, administrators must carry out Task 7, maintaining compliance with employment laws.

■ *Information Management* –
Donna J. Slovensky, PhD, RHIA, FAHIMA, et al.

Six key tasks are identified in the Information Management domain to initiate the process of planning and optimize information resources in the medical practice. To perform Task 1, conducting information systems needs analysis, the administrator must inventory hardware and software resources and identify the information system applications needed to support both the business and clinical functions in a medical practice. Task 2 focuses on facilitating information system procurement and installation to select the right system from among a wide range of products, technologies, and services that are available. Given the considerable financial investment required by the practice to install and upgrade information systems, administrators must understand and carry out the most effective methods for collecting and evaluating vendor proposals.

Once the information system is installed, the medical practice executive must give considerable ongoing attention to Tasks 3, 4, and 5 to ensure optimization of the practice's investment in technology. These tasks involve developing and implementing information system training and support programs, overseeing database management and maintenance, and developing information network security systems, respectively. Key to successful completion of these tasks is the administrator's ability to recruit and maintain staff with the required skills in information technology, formulating database management policies, and designing processes for protecting the physical security of electronic information.

The thrust of Task 6, providing access to electronic education and information resources and systems, is to capitalize on the vast array of available resources to bring training and new knowledge into the practice. Education and information via CD, Internet, and other emerging Web-based technologies can accelerate acquisition of new business and clinical skills in the practice with less impact on work schedules and training budgets than total reliance on the more traditional face-to-face or classroom methodologies. Knowing where to find these resources and how to evaluate them in terms of value and effectiveness are important skills for the practice executive.

■ *Planning and Marketing* –
Reid M. Oetjen, PhD, MSHSA, and Dawn M. Oetjen, PhD, MHA

Planning and marketing have always been important to the growth of a medical practice. From the 1970s and into the 1980s, planning and marketing often were conducted only by large practices. As competition and average practice size increased, planning and marketing became more prevalent. Often misunderstood by both hospitals and medical practices in the 1980s and 1990s, the relationship between planning and marketing (and all of the subsets of marketing such as public relations, advertising, merchandizing, and placement of media) has currently become more understood.

There are six key tasks in this Body of Knowledge domain. Strategically positioning the organization to constantly respond to changes and opportunities in the environment through development of strategic plans is the focus of Task 1. The practice executive must know how to analyze and interpret market research data and guide the planning process to address decisions on mission, vision, goals and objectives; service areas and stakeholder relationships; program, service, and product mix; and competitive advantage.

Through Task 2, using the strategic plan as a foundation, the administrator creates business plans to identify the resources that will be required to achieve goals and determine how they will be appropriately allocated. Because the business plan also serves as a communication tool to gain internal and external stakeholder buy-in, the essential components of the plan and how they should be developed are also part of the administrator's essential knowledge base. Many practices have been successful in reaching out to specific market segments. As a logical outgrowth of the strategic and business plans, Task 3 focuses on the development of marketing plans to formulate strategies responsive to the needs of targeted customer audiences.

Once plans are in place, the emphasis for the administrator shifts to implementation and reporting the results. Task 4, monitoring and evaluating the effectiveness of the strategic, business, and marketing plan activities, requires the administrator to employ a variety of measuring and reporting tools.

Executing market segment initiatives often requires creating external affiliations and partnerships for the practice, which is the thrust of Task 5. Establishing the purpose of the alliance, selecting the best partners, and choosing the appropriate structure are important requirements for success. Finally, the external role of the administrator also manifests itself through Task 6, developing and implementing community outreach as well as public and customer relations programs. The executive must know how to establish trust and demonstrate responsiveness to community needs through program selection and quality.

■ *Professional Responsibility* –
David Peterson, MBA, FACMPE, and Ken Mace, MA, CMPE

Instinctively, most professionals know what professional responsibility means – the responsibilities associated with being a professional. A common body of knowledge, ethical standards, continuing education, peer and self review, academic excellence, and research and publication all contribute to being a professional. This domain entails seven tasks.

Task 1, advancing professional knowledge and leadership skills, addresses the importance of the medical practice executive's ability to assess educational needs and to communicate why it is necessary to plan career advancement. This task places particular emphasis on how to advance the medical practice management profession.

To effectively maintain psychological and physical well-being, Task 2, balancing professional and personal pursuits, addresses the body-mind connection and why health and fitness are integral pats of every successful professional's routine.

Task 3, promoting ethical standards for individual and organizational behavior and decision making, is related to the practice executive's need to develop individual and organizational integrity, and to implement ethical behaviors and goals into the practice's organizational culture. The administrator should set standards for ethical behavior, professionalism, and responsibility to the community, as well as be aware of and communicate the associated risks when ethics are ignored or abused.

Task 4, conducting self-assessments, addresses the administrator's responsibility to identify the programs and resources that are necessary for setting and meeting competency requirements, including professional knowledge and skill assessments and personality classification models. This involves various assessment techniques as well as group and personal dynamics.

The application of knowledge and skills to medical practice management, as well as the ability to share knowledge and information with the profession, are encompassed in Task 5, advancing the profession by contributing to the Body of Knowledge. Examples include perspectives on ambulatory medicine, practice management, community health care, and other health care issues.

The practice executive's knowledge of existing professional organizations and networks, ability to assist people with their next career steps, and coaching and mentoring skills are extremely important. Task 5, engaging in professional networking, addresses how to advance professional advancement through these avenues.

Task 6, developing effective interpersonal skills, focuses on the importance of mastering the presentation of information. Correct verbal and listening skills are the mark of a professional.

■ *Risk Management* –
Geraldine Amori, PhD, ARM, CPHRM

The Risk Management domain includes 11 tasks and encompasses a broad knowledge base that intersects with all other Body of Knowledge domains. Among the many knowledge areas covered in this volume, the ability to draft clear policies and procedures that are designed to mitigate and report risk are integral to the practice executive's role. The responsibility of the board of directors is also encompassed in the development of risk management policies and compliance monitoring, as the practice should continuously assess potential medical practice risks to reduce the possibility of occurrences. This assessment extends beyond malpractice to most areas of the practice in which there is potential risk, such as liability, fraud, and abuse; the Occupational Safety and Health Administration (OSHA); the Health Insurance Portability and Accountability Act of 1996 (HIPAA); and the Employee Retirement Income Security Act of 1974 (ERISA).

At the core of the Risk Management domain is Task 1, the need to maintain legal compliance with the corporate structure of the practice. The ability to carry out this task assumes that the administrator understands federal, state, and local laws, such as antitrust, OSHA and ADA regulations, as well as the board's leadership liability and fiduciary obligations. It also requires the ability to develop and communicate a compliance plan and strategy to others in the practice. Compliance planning and monitoring is broad and includes issues such as physician education, prevention of fraudulent practices, billing errors, record falsification, inadequate documentation of patient care, patient discrimination, client abuse, inadequate safety plans for patients and staff, inadequate reference-checking before hiring, and others.

The compliance plan provides an essential foundation for addressing other tasks to mitigate risk exposure in the practice. Task 2, maintaining the corporate history and developing record-keeping procedures in compliance with applicable laws, can be expedited through use of evolving computer technology. By developing conflict resolution and grievance procedures and appropriate personnel and property security policies in response to Tasks 3 and 5, the administrator provides a platform for addressing employee and employer transactions related to hiring, firing, and other potential employment disputes, such as claims of discrimination, harassment, or unsafe working conditions. Understanding the unique needs of the practice, in terms of exposure and the various types of insurance available to appropriately address them, are prerequisites for performing Task 4, assessing and procuring liability insurance.

The administrator must also address the risks and exposure of the practice related to transactions with patients and various other public entities. Such risks include over- or underutilizing services, patient complaints, and malpractice claims. Having systems in place to assure that the staff monitors and reports situations that result in compromised patient safety, satisfaction, or quality of care is the thrust of Task 6, developing and implementing quality assurance and patient satisfaction programs. The importance of preserving the privacy of patient records has also been elevated by the establishment of regulations such as HIPAA. Task 7 addresses how to establish patient, staff, and organizational confidentiality policies.

Conducting audits and navigating the complexity of the tax code and contracts with private and governmental payers to mitigate financial and legal risk to the practice is the focus of Tasks 8, 10, and 11, which requires considerable attention of the administrator. Having a fundamental understanding of such areas as tax codes, accounting principles, contract provisions, and negotiations will serve the administrator well to manage the daily operations. However, given the constant changes and high degree of specialization required to master all of these areas in the Risk Management domain, the practice and administrator are well advised, through Task 9, to develop professional resource networks for risk-related activities.

Conclusion

THIS SERIES REPRESENTS the desire to continue to add detail and substance to the ACMPE Body of Knowledge. As the reader may know, the *Guide to the Body of Knowledge* is in outline form; the authors who participated in this series understood the importance of elevating the Body of Knowledge outline into a narrative series that would attempt to provide detail and added substance. The authors not only stayed true to the outline of the Body of Knowledge, but added valuable information that conformed to the intent of each of the domains.

The case studies, vignettes, and example questions contained in the volumes further round out the presentation to not only provide knowledge to assist those who are studying for the exams, but also to advance the standing of the Body of Knowledge to a level by which the Body of Knowledge will continue to evolve to becoming a work of literature in and of itself.

The body of knowledge for medical practice executives is an expanding universe that responds to the needs of today's health care organizations. Their job is to help organizations reach objectives through the strategic use of information drawn from the ACMPE Body of Knowledge. The *duty* of medical practice executives is to examine and question the contents of the Body of Knowledge and make new contributions to it.

This collection of work, as a continuously evolving and living representation of the profession, will change and grow over time. Necessary review and modification of the ACMPE Body of Knowledge requires thought, imagination, an awareness of the public interest, and continued research of the role of the medical practice executive.

Notes

1. D. L. Madison, "Notes on the History of Group Practice: The Tradition of the Dispensary," *Medical Group Management Journal* 37, no. 5 (September-October 1990): 52–54, 56–60, 86–93.

2. Ibid.

3. M. K. Gusmano, G. Fairbrother, & H. Park, "Exploring the Limits of the Safety Net: Community Health Centers and Care for the Uninsured," *Health Affairs* 21, no. 6 (2002): 188–194.

4. S. Felt-Lisk, M. McHugh, & E. Howell, "Monitoring Local Safety-Net Providers: Do They Have Adequate Capacity?" *Health Affairs* 21, no. 5 (2002): 277–283.

5. J. S. McAlearney, "The Financial Performance of Community Health Centers, 1996–1999. Clear Evidence That Many CHCs Are on the Brink of Financial Insolvency," *Health Affairs* 21, no. 2 (2002): 219–225.

6. L. Shi, R. M. Politzer, J. Regan, D. Lewis-Idema, & M. Falik, "The Impact of Managed Care on the Mix of Vulnerable Populations Served by Community Health Centers," *Journal of Ambulatory Care Management* 24, no. 1 (2001): 51.

7. B. L. Carlson, J. Eden, D. O'Connor, & J. Regan "Primary Care of Patients without Insurance by Community Health Centers," *Journal of Ambulatory Care Management* 24, no. 2 (2001): 47–59.

8. L. Shi, B. Starfield, J. Xu, R. Politzer, & J. Regan, "Primary Care Quality: Community Health Center and Health Maintenance Organization," *Southern Medical Journal* 96, no. 8 (2003): 787–795.

9. A. S. O'Malley & J. Mandelblatt, "Delivery of Preventive Services for Low-Income Persons over Age 50: A Comparison of Community Health Clinics to Private Doctors' Offices," *Journal of Community Health* 28, no. 3 (2003): 185–197.

10. R. H. Fishbein, "Origins of Modern Premedical Education," *Academic Medicine* 76, no. 5 (2001): 425–429.

11. A. M. Harvey, G. H. Brieger, S. L. Abrams, & V. A. McKusick, "A Model of Its Kind. A Century of Medicine at Johns Hopkins," *The Journal of the American Medical Association* 261, no. 21 (1989): 3136–3142.

12. L. H. Schneck, "Strength in Numbers. Medical Group Practices Fill Vital Niche in U.S. Health Care System," *MGMA Connexion* 4, no. 1 (2004): 31, 34–43.

13. L. S. King, "Medicine in the USA: Historical Vignettes. II. Medical Education: The Early Phases," *Journal of the American Medical Association* 248, no. 6 (1982): 731–734.

14. S. Arbabi, G. J. Jurkovich, F. P. Rivara, et al., "Patient Outcomes in Academic Medical Centers: Influence of Fellowship Programs and In-House On-Call Attending Surgeon," *Archives of Surgery* 138, no. 1 (2003): 47–51; Discussion 51.

15. G. Rosen, *The Structure of American Medical Practice 1875–1941.* (Philadelphia: University of Pennsylvania Press, 1983).

16. W. Knight, *Managed Care: What It Is and How It Works,* 1st ed. (Gaithersburg, Md.: Aspen Publishers, 1998).

17. C. W. Nelson, "Origins of the Private Group Practice of Medicine," *Mayo Clinic Proceedings* 67, no. 3 (1992): 212.

18. C. W. Nelson, "Origins of the Name 'Mayo Clinic'," *Mayo Clinic Proceedings* 72, no. 4 (1997): 296.

19. Schneck, "Strength in Numbers."

20. Ibid.

21. D. R. Smart, *Medical Group Practices in the US: 2004 Edition* (Chicago: American Medical Association, 2004).

22. P. L. Havlicek, *Medical Group Practices in the US: A Survey of Practice Characteristics* (Chicago: American Medical Association, 1999).

23. Smart, *Medical Group Practices in the US: 2004 Edition.*

24. Havlicek, *Medical Group Practices in the US.*

25. Smart, *Medical Group Practices in the US: 2004 Edition.*

26. T. H. Stearns, "How Physicians and Administration Work in Small Groups," *MGM Journal* (May-June 1999).

27. G. Kaplan & S. Patterson, "The Physician Administrator Team: An Optimal Model for Leading Medical Practices," *MGMA Connexion* 1, no. 7 (August 2001).

28. J. Goldsmith, "Hospital/Physician Relationships," *Health Affairs* 12 (1993).

29. D. C. Coddington, K. D. Moore, & E. A. Fischer. "Medical Group Management Assoc.," *Making Integrated Healthcare Work* (1996).

30. J. Kotter, *Leading Change* (Boston: Harvard Business School Press, 1996).

31. J. Kotter, *The Heart of Change* (Boston: Harvard Business School Press, 2002).

32. S. Gabel, *AM NEWS* (December 8, 2003).

33. J. S. Bujak, "Culture in Chaos," *Physician Executive* (May-June 1999).

34. ACMPE, Body of Knowledge, "A Role Delineation Study of Medical Practice Executives" (July 1999).

35. Kaplan & Patterson, "The Physician-Administrator Team."

36. ACMPE, Body of Knowledge, "A Role Delineation Study of Medical Practice Executives" (July 1999).

About the American College of Medical Practices Executives

The American College of Medical Practice Executives (ACMPE), established in 1956, supports and promotes the personal and professional growth of health care leaders to advance the profession of medical practice management. ACMPE is the certification and standard-setting body of the Medical Group Management Association (MGMA), the national membership organization for the medical practice management profession. With more than 4,000 members, ACMPE grants nationally recognized certification and fellowship designations to medical practice executives and leaders. ACMPE developed the industry-standard Body of Knowledge for Medical Practice Management, the foundation for the medical group management industry. The Body of Knowledge serves as the structure for all ACMPE assessments, examinations, and leadership development programs.

Today, ACMPE-certified professionals manage some of the top-performing group practices in the nation and are among the best-compensated for their positions. ACMPE, together with MGMA, provides the resources to support professional development and achievement with services that include mentoring, publications, transcript services, scholarship programs, tutorials, education and professional networking. For more information on ACMPE, go to www.acmpe.com.

About the Author

Lawrence F. Wolper, MBA, FACMPE, is Vice President of Strategic Ventures at Atlantic Health, a large hospital system in northern New Jersey. In that capacity he is responsible for new business ventures in ambulatory care and physician practice. Prior to his current position, for 17 years he was the president of L. Wolper, Inc., in Great Neck, New York, a full-service consulting organization specializing in all aspects of physician group practice, faculty practice, and managed care. In addition, the firm has extensive experience in contract management for large physician group practices and ambulatory surgery centers, as well as practice turn-arounds.

Mr. Wolper has more than 30 years of consulting and senior executive experience, and has been the advisor to, or has managed, major group practices, faculty practice plans, ambulatory surgery centers, and integrated networks. Prior to founding L. Wolper, Inc., in 1987, he was a partner in KPMG, International, LLP, with responsibility, both in New York area and nationwide, for physician practice and ambulatory care consulting. At that time he was involved in the development of large group practices, faculty practice plans, and provider networks. Prior to his partnership in KPMG, he was a consulting partner with Ingram, Weitzman, Mertens & Co., a large regional health care accounting and consulting firm.

He has published over 35 professional journal articles and 7 texts on subjects germane to physician and faculty practice, and to health care administration. His book *Health Care Administration: Principles, Practices, Structure, and Delivery,* Second Edition, won a prestigious national award as one of the top 250 texts in the health sciences industry. He is also managing editor of *Physician Practice Management: Essential Operational and Financial Knowledge,* published by Jones and Bartlett Publishers.

Mr. Wolper received a master of business administration degree in Health Care Administration from Bernard M. Baruch College-Mount Sinai School of Medicine, and a bachelor of arts degree in Advertising/Marketing from Hofstra University. He was a Robert Wood Johnson Foundation Fellow in HMO Management at the Wharton School, University of Pennsylvania, and an Association of University Programs in Hospital Administration (AUPHA) Fellow studying the British National Health System and the Kings Fund College of Hospital Management in London, England.

He is a Fellow in the American College of Medical Practice Executives (ACMPE), and an associate adjunct professor in the Executive MPH Program at Columbia University, teaching a course on managed care and organized delivery systems.